I0437226

25
Ways to Stop
Hair Loss

Annmarie Lloyd

iUniverse, Inc.
Bloomington

25 Ways to Stop Hair Loss

Copyright © 2012 by Annmarie Lloyd

All rights reserved. No part of this book may be used or reproduced by any means, graphic, electronic, or mechanical, including photocopying, recording, taping or by any information storage retrieval system without the written permission of the publisher except in the case of brief quotations embodied in critical articles and reviews.

iUniverse books may be ordered through booksellers or by contacting:

iUniverse
1663 Liberty Drive
Bloomington, IN 47403
www.iuniverse.com
1-800-Authors (1-800-288-4677)

Because of the dynamic nature of the Internet, any web addresses or links contained in this book may have changed since publication and may no longer be valid. The views expressed in this work are solely those of the author and do not necessarily reflect the views of the publisher, and the publisher hereby disclaims any responsibility for them.

Any people depicted in stock imagery provided by Thinkstock are models, and such images are being used for illustrative purposes only.

Certain stock imagery © Thinkstock.

ISBN: 978-1-4759-6127-0 (sc)
ISBN: 978-1-4759-6128-7 (e)

Printed in the United States of America

iUniverse rev. date: 11/14/2012

DEDICATION

This to dedicates to my family, clients and staff of Annmarie Hair Care, who are so dear to me with their support, love, hope, encouragement and faithful commitment of my work in the hair care industry.

Contents

ACKNOWLEDGEMENT

I want to take this opportunity to thank my Savior and my Lord He gave me wisdom in all things. To my family, friends and clients who I have been their hair care expert over twenty four years in the beauty Industry. To Karl Richmond with him in seminars and workshops I have learnt products knowledge and to Dr. Sandra Gilman who taught hair loss, Scalp disorders and its care from the elan center for trichology.

A special thank to Melissa Bogdany for her editorial assistance and prepared the format of this book and thank to iUniverse publisher and their team also for their editorial assistance and publishing this book. Thank you all.

What Is Hair Loss?

Hair loss is the effect of some conditions, such as brittle hair, hair breakage, hair shedding, thinning hair, alopecia, short hair syndrome, and various other disorders. Causes include the misuse of chemicals, excessive heat applications, bonding glue, tight weaves, tight braids, and a wide array of maladies. Some conditions can be temporarily treated by trichologists and dermatologists.

This book will teach you how to avoid and stop the problem before it cannot be permanently repaired. Common sense is used when identifying the problem and seeking help from a trichologist or dermatologist. Therefore, you will find this book very useful in addressing this issue.

Introduction

All types of hair—whether it is virgin (not chemically treated), is natural, is processed with permanent curl, is chemically treated, or is straightened with a hot comb—can and will experience hair loss. Most people don't pay attention to the problem until they start to lose hair. Then, they seek the cause of the hair loss.

To determine whether you will experience hair loss, you will need to see a trichologist (hair and scalp specialist). A trichologist does consultation, diagnosis, etiology, and prognosis, and recommends treatment of your hair and scalp. Trichologists work closely with other professionals, including medical doctors, internal specialists, psychiatrists, dermatologists, dentists, nutritionists, endocrinologists, family practitioners, and other trichologists. They also teach and advise on the care of your hair and scalp. It is very important to keep up with your visits to the trichologist and prevent further damage down the road.

Before your visit to the beauty salon to receive a chemical treatment or any other procedure, such as a braid, weave, or bonding style, seek the advice and consultation of a trichologist. Hopefully, you'll find you have healthy hair and learn many ways to prevent or stop hair loss.

1

Avoid Buildup on the Hair and Scalp

Some hair products can leave buildup on the scalp. This can cause the scalp pores and hair follicles to become clogged, which can cause hair growth to cease temporarily. These products include hair spray, extreme hair grease, and styling mousse. In addition, unclean hair can lead to buildup. These things also can cause dryness on the scalp, or contact dermatitis. This dryness, which can take a long time to clear up, causes the scalp to itch. As a result of scratching, you may irritate the scalp and peel the epidermal layer, pulling the hair out from the root. Constantly doing this causes short hair syndrome.

SOLUTION: Shampoo hair weekly, ensuring the scalp and hair remain clean and healthy. When hair loss occurs, treat the scalp as suggested by a trichologist or dermatologist after your consultation and examination. If the scalp is irritated or sore, seek the help of a dermatologist or medical doctor, who may recommend medication to treat it. Avoid buildup in the future, as it may cause permanent hair loss.

2

Shampoo and Treat the
Hair and Scalp Weekly

A dirty scalp creates a home for disease (bacteria) that can affect hair growth as well as cause aging damage to the scalp. When that occurs, it causes itching. When you scratch, you tear the layer of the epidermal cells, causing irritation and tenderness to the scalp. Underneath the skin, bacteria breed, and the hair follicles become inflamed because of the growing bacteria. An interruption of hair growth causes disorders called folliculitis hair loss and scarring alopecia.

SOLUTION: Shampoo the hair at least once a week to maintain healthy hair and a healthy scalp. A trichologist or dermatologist will recommend treatment for scalp irritation and sores that will heal the tenderness of the scalp, recently scratched. A regular scalp treatment by your trichologist will help promote a healthy scalp.

3

Never Allow the Chemical to Sit on the Hair and Scalp Long to Straighten Hair

When you attempt to get your hair straight by leaving the chemical relaxer on the hair and scalp, the hair gets overprocessed and the scalp burns. The new growth also gets processed while in the hair follicle because the chemical relaxer penetrates the scalp for a long period of time. So when the eight to twelve weeks are up and it's time for a retouch, you can't see the virgin hair because it is already processed. Trying to reprocess the hair will cause overprocessing of the hair and damage the scalp, resulting in traction hair loss.

SOLUTION: Always base the scalp with protector shield before applying relaxer to the hair and new growth. Never leave relaxer on the hair for more than five to ten minutes. The hair must be 75 to 85 percent straight to maintain healthy hair, as hair is already fragile. It is not necessary to overprocess the hair. When that does occur, seek help from a trichologist or dermatologist, who will analyze the hair and prescribe the best treatment for the condition of your hair and scalp.

Apply the Chemical Only to the New Growth of the Previously Relaxed Hair

Processed hair or previously relaxed hair does not need repeated straightening because that eventually will cause overprocessing. During overprocessing, the hair begins to shed and break away, resulting in short hair alopecia. When hair is relaxed, it becomes permanently changed and is fragile, so it will become overprocessed if the chemical relaxer is applied repeatedly. Hair breaks away and will result in hair loss, and the result will be no hair left on your head.

SOLUTION: If your hair is already breaking, remove the chemical service, trim off all damaged hair, and focus on repairing the hair. If it has been previously relaxed and is in good condition, apply to the new growth. Otherwise, seek the advice of a trichologist. He or she will advise you to maintain hair and scalp care, and your hairstylist will give the practical instruction on regular visits. Please keep your hairstylist updated at all times to gain healthy hair and a healthy scalp.

5

Never Apply Permanent Curl (Thio) on Sodium Hydroxide-Processed Hair

Hair that is processed with sodium hydroxide is fragile and cannot have another alkaline chemical, such as permanent curl (ammonia thio), applied to it. Doing so is called twin attacking, and during this all the hair becomes breakable and cut away until there is no more hair on the head. When the hair is cut off, there is no curl in the hair that you have desired from the permanent curl. It slowly takes all of your hair, which is called traction hair loss.

SOLUTION: You have two options: Either you wear chemical relaxer (sodium hydroxide) or permanent curl (ammonia thio), such as Jheri curl, dry curl, or wave. You cannot have both, as both chemical treatments together can damage hair completely. To wear chemical relaxer, handle it with care by your hair stylist. A trichologist can analyze, diagnose, and determine the problem that needs to be treated. Wear permanent curl hair in various styles, and never apply sodium hydroxide to the curled hair. Trim hair ends once a month, apply a deep conditioner treatment on every chemical treatment, and apply leave-in treatment after each shampoo to maintain healthy hair.

6

Never Braid Hair Too Tight

Braiding hair is common in various styles, such as plait, cornrow, or twist, but when braiding the hair too tight in an attempt to keep the braid longer, the tight braids will pull the hair out from the roots, causing damage to the scalp and headaches. When this happens, it means the hair is being pulled too tight. Then, slowly the hair falls out, causing hair loss.

SOLUTION: To loosen the tension, try braiding hair one-eighth of an inch away from the scalp. Never pull hair up to attempt to get the maximum tension. The scalp does not move up too close to the braid when doing a plait, cornrow, or twist. The braid must be loose to promote a healthy scalp, which leads to a healthy head of hair.

7

Never Sew in a Weave Too Tight

Sewing weave technique has similar problems to braiding. When people want the weave to stay in their hair longer, they don't understand that sewing it too tight will cause hair loss, which can be permanent, and can damage the scalp. The tight weave causes the hair to pull out from the roots, and slowly you begin to lose a lot of hair and notice your hair is thinner. When wearing the hair weave and not having it shampooed, the hair that is dirty will cause infection on the scalp. The infection can cause constant itching and folliculitis hair loss.

SOLUTION: It is easy to cornrow the base hair a little loose before sewing on the hair weave. While sewing on the hair weave, never pull the thread around the braid too tight, and shampoo the hair and scalp weekly to promote healthy hair and a healthy scalp, and to prevent dryness and itching on the scalp. A trichologist will recommend treatment for dryness and itching on the scalp for all types of braids.

8

Never Use a Broken-Toothed Comb on the Hair and Scalp

Combing the hair removes tangles and nicely styles the hair in various ways. However, never use a broken-toothed comb, as it would tear and split the hair. It can cause constant splitting of the hair, and then it can break away the hair shaft, and you will no longer have the layer to protect the inner structure of the hair. Sometimes it causes twists in the hair and permanently damages the hair. The hair would be difficult to repair, leading to severe hair splitting and breakage (trichoptilosis).

SOLUTION: Throw away your broken-toothed combs, and replace them with a new, flexible comb. When a comb gets worn and cracks, throw it away and replace it with a new one to keep the hair from splitting, becoming brittle, and breaking. If you do this, you will notice your head's full of healthy hair all the time.

9

Never Use a Damaged
Brush on Your Hair

Brushing the hair helps style it in various ways, but using a damaged brush will cause hair damage similar to that caused by using a broken-toothed comb. Some hairbrushes can cause pulling and uprooting of the hair. Brushing wet or damp hair will cause hair splitting and breaking that cannot be repaired, as well as constant shedding of the hair, which can lead to short hair syndrome and trichoptilosis.

SOLUTION: There are various types of hairbrushes for a variety of uses. For a healthy brushing, use a wide-space vent brush with a flexible rubber base and ball tips on the bristles and a natural bristle brush. Throw away all damaged and old brushes. Furthermore, follow the hair-brushing instructions of the trichologist and cosmetologist.

10

Never Apply Permanent Color Right After Rinsing Out Chemical Relaxer

When you chemically relax your hair, and you want beautiful color to brighten your look, never apply the permanent color right after you have rinsed the chemical relaxer from your hair. As you know, chemical relaxer contains sodium hydroxide, which is high alkaline that permanently changes the natural curl pattern. When adding another alkaline chemical (double attacking), it cuts the hair off completely, and sometimes hair slowly shed until you have no hair left; the result is a loss of hair.

SOLUTION: It is best you visit your hairstylist for a professional coloring and chemical relaxing service. The hairstylist will advise you to permanently color your hair two to three weeks before or after receiving chemical relaxer. Always deep condition your hair to maintain healthy hair at all times.

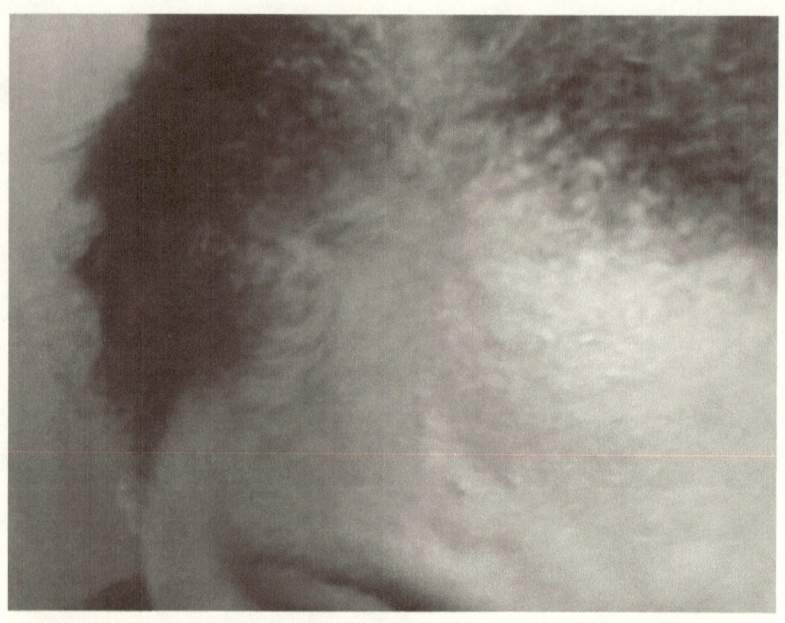

Thinning hairline caused by constant wearing braiding & weaving over the years

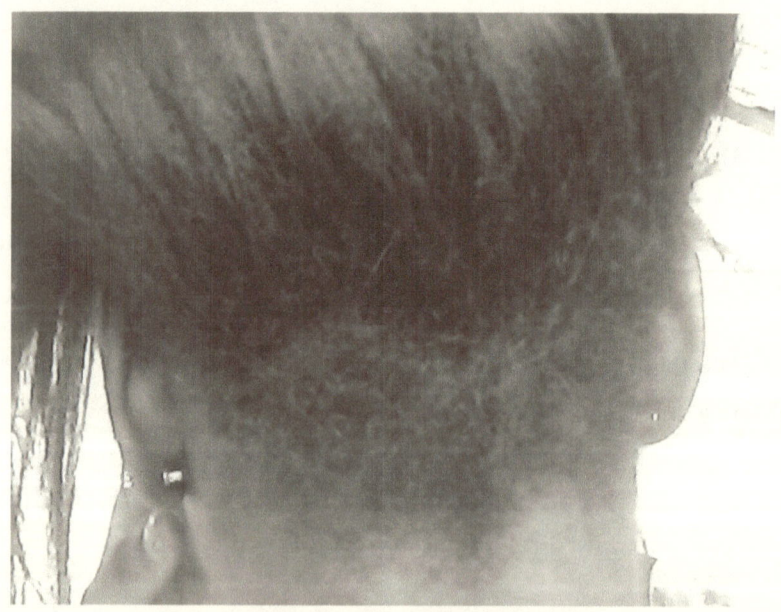

Traction hair loss caused over-processed of chemical relaxer not being rinsed out properly

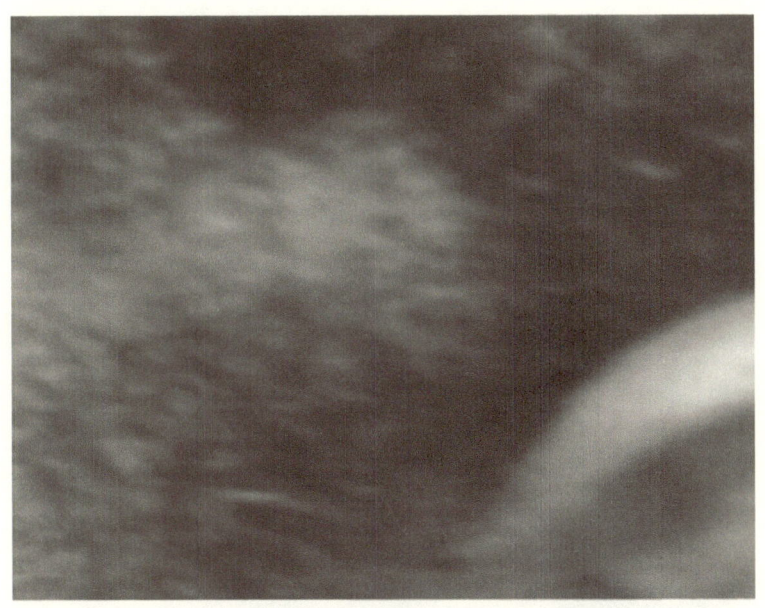

Thinning hairline above the ear caused constant wearing tight braiding for years

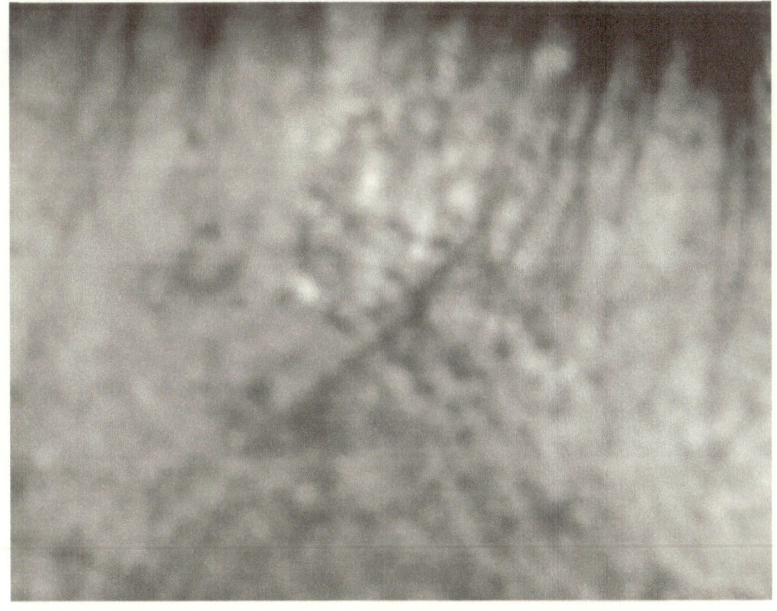

Scarring alopecia caused by constant scalp burns of chemical relaxer

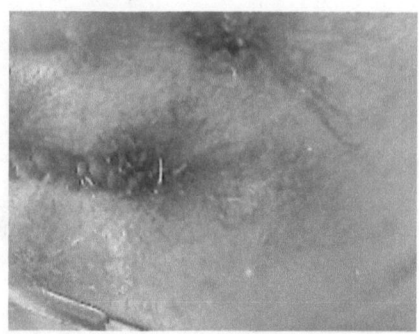

This is traction hairloss caused by excessive tight braids

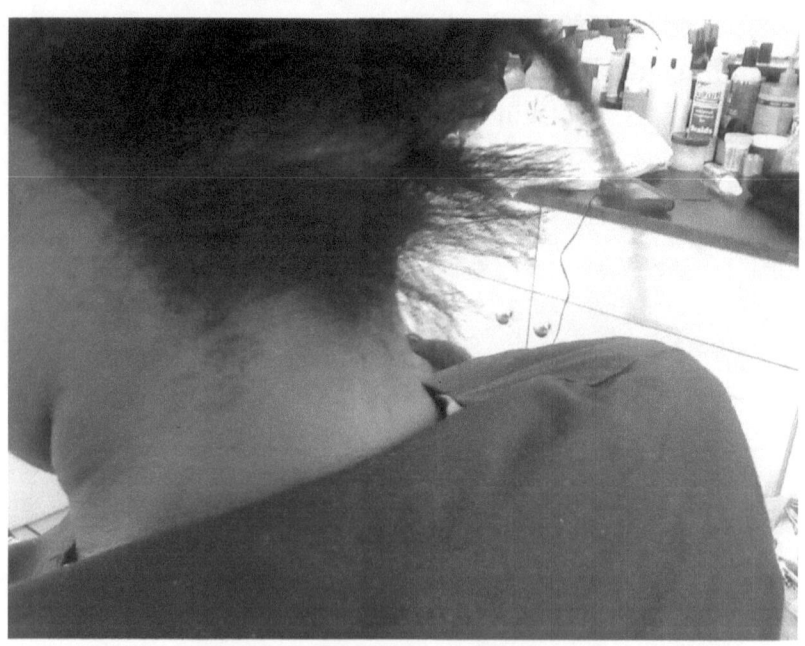

caused by tight braids, tight sew in, take down
& relaxed same day

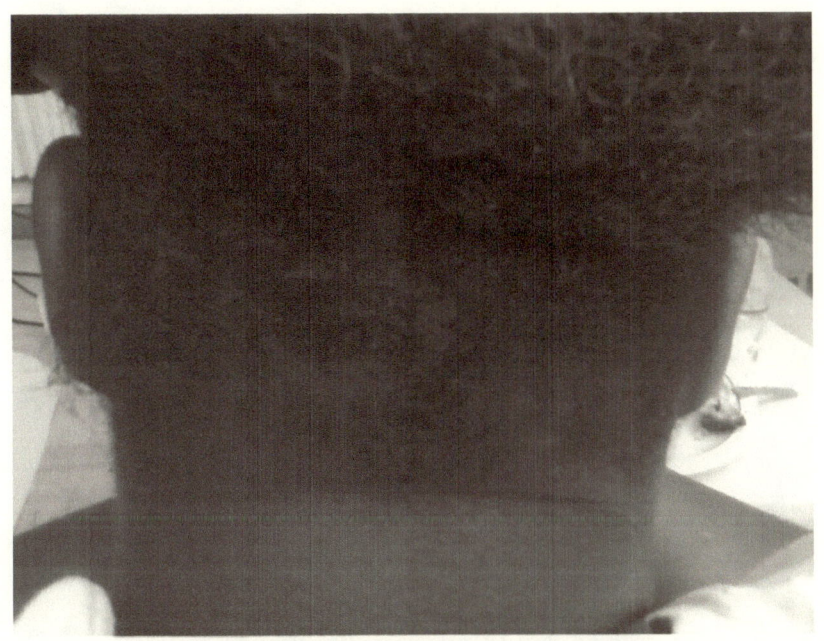

caused by over-processed of relaxer

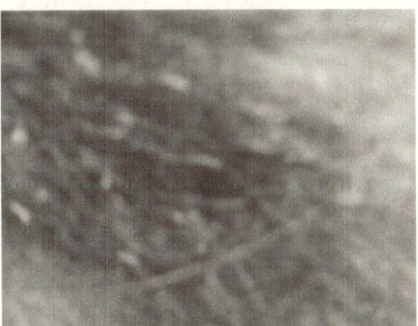

Many years of wearing tight braids, weave and same day
relaxer after taking down extension, scar tissue confirmed
hair will never grow back permanent

11

Never Apply Sodium Hydroxide Relaxer on Permanently Curled Hair

You never want to apply sodium hydroxide relaxer on hair with permanent curl. Doing so will cut off your permanently curled hair. The hair begins to look too dry, becomes brittle, and breaks away. You have to choose whether you want to have your hairstylist give you permanently curled hair or sodium hydroxide-relaxed hair. You will love it when you make your own choice to have either permanent curl or sodium hydroxide-relaxed hair.

SOLUTION: For a sodium hydroxide-relaxed hairstyle, always deep condition the hair, trim ends of hair every month, and keep hair lubricated at all times. For permanent curl hairstyles, get your hair trimmed once a month, recondition, and apply protein to maintain healthy hair at all times.

12

Never Apply Permanent Curl to Pressed Hair

Pressed hair straightening by a hot comb leaves hair temporarily straight, it weakens the hair strands, it means 50 percent of the curl pattern has been removed, and the hair is no longer 100 percent virgin. Therefore, adding a chemical, such as permanent curl, will cut the hair off and leave it lifeless, dull, and brittle. Then, the hair will not penetrate the ammonia acid chemical inside the hair structure, and the hair will not curl and be smooth. Slowly the hair begins to break away, until you see dull hair and thinning.

SOLUTION: Pressed hair needs to be cut off, and you have to wait until the hair grows to full virgin hair before receiving the permanent curl within six to twelve months. Bear in mind that hair grows half an inch every month, and you must see sufficient hair growth before the hair is ready to receive a chemical service.

13

Never Wind the Hair on Rollers Too Tight and Close to the Scalp

Rollers are used to form curly, wavy, or straight hairstyles. However, winding the hair on rollers too tight and close to the scalp, or pulling the hair roots up close to the rollers will cause damage to the scalp, and the constant pulling and struggling while winding the hair on rollers will cause severe hair breakage, especially around the hairline and the nape of the neck. Those are the weaker spots, where hair breaks and gets damaged more easily.

SOLUTION: Try to loosen the rollers, especially around the hairline and the nape of the neck. Do not wind the rollers too tight. If possible, wrapping the hair is best. Loosen and prevent tension of the hair wound on the rollers. If you already lose hair around the hairline, nape of the neck, and crown area, see a trichologist, who will recommend treatment to ensure growth of the hair.

14

Be Careful to Keep Hair
Away From Fire

Most hair products are flammable, and the buildup of those products will catch fire easily. This can cause not only significant hair loss, but also scalp inflammation. This hair will never grow back. Sometimes this causes constant shedding and is difficult to repair. The heat from the flame and smoke causing the shedding of hair results in scarring and cicatricial hair loss.

SOLUTION: Be careful to keep your hair away from open flames, lit tobacco products, other fires, or sparks. Cover your hair with a hair wrap while working in the kitchen at your home or at a restaurant. Shampoo your hair weekly to reduce the risk of it igniting.

15

Always Cover Hair While Cooking

Excessive heat from fire tends to damage the hair, especially when you're working in the kitchen or a restaurant, or doing heavy construction work. When hair is exposed to this environment, the hair will begin shedding and break away. Treating the hair weekly and returning to the same environment with heat will not prevent damage or help repair the hair. Instead, the hair will always shed and break away, or you will be left with no hair, or temporary hair loss.

SOLUTION: Whether or not your hair is clean, cover your hair with a hair net or a bouffant cap to keep the hair from being damaged in an environment with heat. This will help you maintain healthy hair, free of shedding and breakage, and prevent hair loss.

16

While a Chemical Relaxer Is on the Hair, Never Place It Under a Hair Dryer

Chemical hair relaxers have heat active in them during processing, and placing hair with a chemical relaxer on it under a heated hair dryer to speed the process can cause serious burn and permanent damage to the hair and scalp. Chemicals include sodium hydroxide and ammonium thioglycolate, among others. They are powerfully acidic and alkaline, can cause inflammation of the scalp and hair loss, and are dangerous to your health, possibly even causing death.

SOLUTION: Follow the manufacturer's instructions for a proper procedure, and avoid future damage to your hair and scalp. Visit a trichologist for consultation to ensure you have a healthy scalp and head of hair.

17

Always Use a Neutralizing Shampoo or Stabilizer After Each Chemical Relaxer Service

After rinsing out the relaxer and shampooing the hair without the neutralizing shampoo or stabilizer, the action of the chemical relaxer continues to activate the hair. That causes shedding to begin and the hair to become dry, dull, and brittle. You wonder why the hair is breaking away, after you did rinse out the relaxer, shampoo the hair, and apply treatment. Remember, regular shampoo does not stop the action of the relaxer, and without the use of a stabilizer, the hair will experience shedding.

SOLUTION: After rinsing out all traces of chemical relaxer, a neutralizing shampoo is required to prevent further action of the chemical on the hair and bring it down to its normal pH. Using a stabilizer can balance the hair to its normal pH and will help promote healthy hair at all times. A professional hairstylist must follow the proper steps and use a stabilizer or neutralizing shampoo.

18

A Chemical Service on Natural (Virgin) Hair That Has Been Frequently Blown Dry Is Not Recommended

Natural (virgin) hair that has been frequently blown dry, after each shampoo, is easily straight, as the heat from the blow-dryer removes 25 to 50 percent of the natural curl from the hair, temporarily straightening it. This hair is fragile. When this hair is chemically treated, the relaxer causes the hair to be doubly processed, which will cause constant splitting and breaking, and the hair will be difficult to repair. The result will be hair loss.

SOLUTION: To keep your hair 100 percent virgin, never apply heat from a blow-dryer or underneath a hood dryer. Use low or cool drying to dry the excess water from the hair so the hair will not be heat-processed, and then the hair qualifies to receive a chemical treatment, and you will have healthy, chemically treated hair.

19

Never Blow-Dry Permanently Curled Hair to Make It Straight

Permanent curl is also fragile, and it swells when applying the first step (rearranger). That chemical opens up the cuticle; that's why waving lotion (booster) is applied—to close up the cuticle while it re-forms and the curl sets before applying neutralizer solution to tighten the curl. But in blow-drying the permanent curl after each shampoo, the heat will penetrate and help open the cuticle, and also split it open. The split causes dryness, brittleness, and breaking away of the hair—and these things result in hair loss.

SOLUTION: After each shampoo, towel-dry the hair, but do not use heat from a blow-dryer or hood dryer. That's the way permanent curl must be handled before applying the gel activator and moisturizer to keep the hair lubricated and prevent dullness, dryness, and brittleness. Do this, and you will have durable, healthy hair.

20

Never Add Tension on Ponytail Hairstyles

Ponytail hairstyles are good-looking in various fashions, but adding too much tension to the scalp by pulling the hair, forcing it to be smooth and neat will cause breakage, a tearing away of the hair shaft, and permanent damage to the scalp, which is traction hair loss, especially around the hairline, nape of the neck, and crown area of the head. Sometimes the hair never grows back.

SOLUTION: When doing a ponytail hairstyle, do not add tension to the hair, but always loosen the hair to prevent further damage to the hair and scalp. Also, do not wear ponytail hairstyles frequently, which would cause weighing on the scalp and hair. Then, you will see healthy hair.

21

Never Use Chemical Relaxer as a Substitute for Hair Glue Remover

If you attempt to remove a hair weave and bonding glue from your hair by using chemical relaxer as a substitute for bonding glue remover, the hair tears. And forcing out the bonding glue with a comb while the relaxer is on the hair causes overprocessing of the hair and tearing of the outer hair (cuticle layer) from the hair strand. In constantly doing this, with every removal of a weave and bonding glue from the hair, you're tearing and irritating the scalp, causing folliculitis hair loss. The scalp becomes smooth and permanently bald.

SOLUTION: Never apply bonding glue on the scalp. Only apply the glue on the hair root one-fourth of an inch away from the scalp so the bonding glue won't penetrate the scalp and cause any permanent damage. Always use bonding glue remover on glue to soften it so it will be easy to remove, without damaging the hair and scalp. Then you can have healthy hair and a healthy scalp.

22

Never Apply Too Much Heat
on Glued Scalp and Hair

Many people apply excessive heat from a blow-dryer on the bonding weave to ensure the weave stays on the hair firmly. The heat along with bonding infects the scalp, causing scarring scalp disorders when wearing the heated bonding weave at each service and replacing after taking down the weave constantly. You are asking for folliculitis hair loss.

SOLUTION: When bonding the hair weave on your natural hair, try using low heat for thirty seconds. The bond will stay. Shampoo the hair regularly for cleansing and a healthy scalp. After taking down the hair weave, wait seven to fourteen days before reapplying the bonding weave to your hair to prevent scalp disorder, hair shedding, and hair breakage.

23

Never Reapply Chemical Relaxer on the Hair Another Day After a Chemical Service

If the hair has not been properly straightened the day before and you attempt to reapply the relaxer to the hair to ensure proper straightening, it will cause the hair to be overprocessed. The hair begins to experience shedding and breaks slowly until you have the hair cut off. You will have difficulty repairing that condition, and the result is temporary hair loss.

SOLUTION: When the hair is not properly processed, wait six weeks before you get a retouch. That way you can prevent hair loss. Before you apply the relaxer on the hair, analyze the hair to determine its condition, texture, and porosity so you know which strength and type of relaxer should be used on your hair to give you straight and healthy hair.

24

Do Not Place Permanently Curled Hair That Is Rodded With Booster Under a Hair Dryer

Permanent curl (Jheri curl), the curl booster, contains ammonium thioglycolate and other chemical ingredients that close the cuticle of the hair after rinsing out the curl relaxer (which rises and opens up the cuticle), bringing the hair to its normal balance while it's being rodded. But placing the hair under a heated hair dryer helps the curl booster chemical penetrate the hair follicles, and it gets trapped inside, causing folliculitis, scarring alopecia, hair thinning, and traction hair loss.

SOLUTION: The manufacturer did not state that you need to place hair that is rodded with curl booster under a hair dryer. Do not place permanently curled hair that is rodded with curl booster under a heated hair dryer. Instead, place the hair under a plastic cap, and follow the manufacturer's instructions. Leave the cap on for ten to thirty minutes, and then rinse out with tap water for five to fifteen minutes. Then, blot the hair dry using a towel. Then, saturate the rods with curl neutralizer, leave it on for five to fifteen minutes, according to the manufacturer's instructions. Then, rinse for five minutes, remove the rods, and proceed to style.

25

Never Sew in or Braid Hair the Same Day After Chemically Treated

As you already know, chemically treated hair is fragile and breaks easily. After rinsing out the chemical relaxer, hair is shampooed and dried. Then you proceed to sew in or braid the hair with extension hair. This weakens the hair strands, and slowly the hair breaks. In doing this procedure, you will experience thinning hair and scalp, resulting in hair loss.

SOLUTION: After chemically treating the hair, wait at least seven to fourteen days before getting a sew-in or braid with extension hair. Then, the hair is in good condition to receive that procedure, and it prevents hair breakage and thinning hair and scalp. You will have long-lasting, healthy hair and a healthy scalp.

Conclusion

There are many ways to stop hair loss, and it is very easy to follow the steps to prevent it if you are willing to make the sacrifice and obey the instructions, take the precautions, and do the right things.

As you know, hair is fragile, and even more so when it has received a chemical service. Therefore, hair needs the proper maintenance each day. You should seek the help of professional hairstylists, trichologists, and dermatologists. When you have patience and are educated about the proper procedures, you will enjoy healthy hair.

References

www.Annmariehaircare.com

About the Author

Annmarie Lloyd, a beauty salon owner, has worked in beauty salons since 1988. She has been a salon owner for more than twenty years. Below you can read more about her accomplishments in the industry:

1988: Awarded Most Outstanding Student, Lister Mair/Gilby School for the Deaf; Awarded Most Outstanding Student, Leon's School of Beauty Culture

1988-89: Hard worker at three beauty salons

1993-2000: Member of the National Association of Hairdressers and Cosmetologists (NAHC)

1996-2000: Chairperson of NAHC

1988-2008: Attended seminars and workshops

2008: Awarded Most Outstanding Student, The Elan Center for Trichology (TECT); became certified trichologist (hair and scalp care specialist)

2009: Became a presenter for trichology seminars

1990-present: Beauty salon owner

www.ingramcontent.com/pod-product-compliance
Lightning Source LLC
Chambersburg PA
CBHW050346290526
45785CB00006B/2656